COOKBOOK FOR PARKINSON'S DISEASE NUTRITION

Nutritional advice for Parkinson's disease sufferers

DR. CRAIG CONNER

Table of Contents

CHAPER ONE

Parkinson's Disease Nutrition

Nutritional advice for Parkinson's disease sufferers

If you have Parkinson's disease, you don't need to follow a special diet. In addition, the stiffness or difficulty controlling your body movements can make it difficult for you to eat healthily. To maintain your strength and keep your

Parkinson's meds working as they should, you'll need to eat a diet rich in vitamins and minerals.

Many people with Parkinson's suffer from weight loss, difficulty swallowing, and gastrointestinal issues as a result of medication. A registered dietitian or your primary care physician may be able to help you deal with these issues.

Cooking and Eating a Healthy Diet

Make sure to eat a wide variety of foods from each food group. Check with your doctor first if you think you need vitamin supplements.

Exercise and a healthy diet can help you maintain a healthy weight for your age and height.

A diet rich in fruits, vegetables, and whole-grain foods can help you lose weight and keep it off.

Consume fewer calories by cutting back on sugar, salt, saturated fats found in meat and dairy products, and cholesterol.

Every day, drink eight cups of water.

Ask your doctor if you're allowed to drink. Some medications may not work properly as a result.

Drugs and food should be taken together.

Parkinson's disease is best treated with levodopa. Ideally, you should take it 30 minutes before or one hour after a meal, depending on your preference. However, some people may experience nausea as a result.

Even if your doctor prescribes something else, the nausea may not go away on its own. That's why, if you're experiencing side effects, your doctor may recommend that you take medication.

Ask your doctor if cutting back on protein is necessary. Levodopa may not work as well if you eat a lot of protein.

Get Rid of Vomiting

Try these tips to avoid or alleviate nausea:

Clear or icy-cold beverages are best. Sugary drinks may soothe your stomach more effectively than water.

Keep away from orange and grapefruit juices and other acidic drinks.

Slowly savor each sip.

Instead of consuming liquids during meals, drink them between them.

Consume simple foods such as saltine crackers or plain bread in order to avoid overindulgence.

Avoid foods that are fried, greasy, or sugary.

Slowly savor each mouthful and eat more frequently.

Don't mix hot and cold food together..

Avoid getting sick from the smell of hot or warm foods by eating cold or room-temperature foods.

After a meal, take a few minutes to relax but keep your head up. You may vomit as a result of physical activity.

Brushing your teeth after a meal is a bad idea.

Before getting out of bed, eat some crackers if you're feeling nauseous. Try a protein-rich snack like lean meats or cheese before going to bed.

When you're not feeling so sick, it's best to eat.

CHAPTER TWO

Drinking or Mouth Dryness

This can be a side effect of some Parkinson's medications. There are a number of things you can do to alleviate your pain:

Do not go a day without drinking at least 8 cups of water Some Parkinson's sufferers may also have heart issues and may need to monitor their fluid intake. Consult your physician for advice on how much fluid you should consume.

Reduce the amount of caffeine in your diet by limiting your intake of caffeine-rich beverages like coffee, tea, cola and chocolate.

Breads, toast, cookies, and crackers can all be softened. Decaffeinated tea and coffee can also be used as a dip.

Take a sip of water after every bite of food to help you swallow.

Adding sauces to food will soften and moisten it, thus making it more enjoyable. Cooking with butter is a great way to add flavor to your food.

To increase saliva production and moisten your mouth, try eating sour candy or fruit ice.

Avoid most mouthwashes because they often contain alcohol, which can cause drying of the mouth and other oral health problems. Find out if there is anything else you can do from your doctor or dentist.

Obtain prescription artificial saliva from your doctor.

While tired, it is best to avoid eating.

It's possible that you won't have enough energy later in the day to eat a full meal.

Save your energy for eating by preparing simple foods. Involve your family in meal preparation if you're staying with them.

Consider using a courier service. Some supermarkets carry them. Check with your local Meals on Wheels program to see if you qualify for free or low-cost food delivery.

Be sure to stock up on healthy snacks like fresh fruits and vegetables or high-fiber cold cereals.

When you're feeling drained, grab a frozen portion of your meal and heat it up when you're hungry again.

Take a break before eating to make the most of your meal. Eat your largest meal of the day first thing in the morning to give your body the energy it needs for the rest of the day.

When You Don't Have a Stomach.

You may not feel like eating at all on some days.

Talk to your doctor about your situation. Depression has been linked to a decreased desire to eat certain foods. When you receive treatment, you can expect your appetite to return.

Make yourself hungry by taking a walk or engaging in some other light activity.

Don't overeat by drinking liquids after you've finished your meal.

Put your personal favorites on the menu. Start with the heaviest, most caloric items on your plate. Avoid sugary sodas, candy, and chips, however.

Try new foods and ingredients to spice up your meals.

Snack on high-protein, high-calorie options such as these:

- Ice cream.

- Cheese

- Bars of granola

- Custard

- Sandwiches

With cheese, nachos are even better.

- Eggs

- Peanut butter crackers

• Half-and-half cereal

• Yogurt made from Greek yoghurt

Maintain a Proper Body Mass Index

Parkinson's patients frequently suffer from malnutrition and weight loss. So, keeping tabs on your weight is a smart idea.

Unless your doctor instructs you otherwise, weigh yourself no more than once or twice a week. Diuretics and steroids, such as prednisone, should be weighed every day if you're taking them.

Any significant weight gain or loss (more than 2 pounds per day) should be addressed by you and/or your physician. In order to keep your condition under control, they may suggest dietary adjustments.

If you'd like to put on weight, this is the place to look.

Consult your physician to determine whether or not nutritional supplements are appropriate for you to take.

Some of these can be harmful or interfere with your medication.

Keep away from low-fat and low-calorie foods unless you've been specifically instructed to eat them. Instead, use full-fat milk, full-fat cheese, and full-fat yogurt instead.

Practicing a healthy diet

The best way to eat when you have Parkinson's disease is to eat a healthy, well-balanced diet that includes plenty of fruits and vegetables.

Eating foods rich in antioxidants is one way to maintain a healthy weight. Tobacco smoke, air pollution, and the metabolic process of turning food into energy are just a few of the stresses that these "good for you" molecules help protect cells from. Several foods and beverages, including dark chocolate and red wine, are rich in antioxidants.

CHAPTER THREE

Using Food as Medicine to Relieve Symptoms

The first step in treating some Parkinson's symptoms is to alter your diet.

Regularity can be maintained by consuming more fluids and consuming more fiber. You should drink at least six to eight 8-ounce glasses of water each day. Drinking warm liquids, especially in the morning, can help you get your bowels moving. Fruits, vegetables, legumes, and whole grain breads and cereals are all good sources of fiber in the diet, as is the peel from fruits and vegetables. Additionally, the majority of these foods are high in anti-inflammatory antioxidants.

Increase fluid and salt intake to raise blood pressure, but check with your doctor first, especially if you have heart or kidney problems. Water and saltier drinks like Gatorade and V8 juice can be used as fluids. Caffeine and alcohol can dehydrate and lower blood pressure, so limit their use. Blood pressure fluctuations can be minimized by eating small, frequent meals.

Speak to a speech therapist if you're having trouble swallowing (coughing, choking, or food feeling "stuck"). Altering your diet to make it easier to swallow could include softening your food or including foods that do just that (such as seasoned, sour or carbonated foods). Taking smaller bites at a slower pace, or tucking your chin to your chest when you swallow, are examples of techniques that can help you eat more slowly.

-

Muscle cramps can be alleviated by consuming turmeric-infused yellow mustard or tonic water, both of which contain the anti-inflammatory compound quinine. Others swear by the use of salt, vinegar, or pickle juice. Consistent hydration may lessen or eliminate cramping.

Consult a doctor or a dietitian to develop a diet that will help you manage the symptoms of

Parkinson's disease while also making you feel healthy and energised.

Medication and Dietary Changes

There are many proteins that compete for absorption, and levodopa (Sinemet) is one of them. Meat and fish, which are high in protein, may reduce the amount of levodopa that enters your system and the effectiveness of a dose. Taking levodopa at mealtime may not be a problem if your symptoms are mild early on in your disease. Taking your medication 30 minutes before or 60 minutes after a meal may be an option if your medication isn't working as well as it should or if it wears off before your next dose. It's also possible to save higher protein intake for the end of the day, when symptom control isn't as urgently needed.

Levodopa absorption can be reduced by taking iron supplements. At least two hours before or after taking levodopa, take these medications.

Levodopa is found in faba beans, making them a good candidate for inclusion in a healthy diet. Unfortunately, the levodopa content of fava beans is unknown, and it is likely that it is very low.

Pramipexole, ropinirole, and rotigotine are dopamine agonists that don't necessitate any dietary changes. If you're taking MAO-B inhibitors (rasagaline and selegiline) and eating foods high in tyramine, you may see an increase in blood pressure. You don't have to cut out these foods completely from your diet,

but you should consume them in
moderation.

THE END